PCOS DIET COOKBOOK
FOR FERTILITY

Nourishing Your Way to Fertility and Wellness with 150 Delicious Recipes and Expert Guidance.

Willow Monroe

"You are about to go on a trip that has the potential to alter the course of your life and give you more control as you make your way toward becoming a parent. This cookbook is more than simply a collection of dishes; rather, it is your reliable travel companion on the path toward controlling polycystic ovary syndrome (PCOS) and boosting your fertility."

DISCLAIMER

Every effort has made this book as complete and accurate as possible. This book provides information only up to the publishing date. Therefore, this book should be used as a guide, not the ultimate source.

The purpose of this book is to educate. The author and the publisher do not warrant that the information contained in this book is fully complete and shall not be responsible for any errors or omissions. The author and publisher shall have neither liability nor responsibility to any person or entity concerning any loss or damage caused or alleged to be caused directly or indirectly by this book.

Table Of Content

Introduction

As you approach parenthood, you are about to engage on a journey that could potentially alter the course of your life and provide you with greater autonomy. Beyond being a mere compilation of recipes, this cookbook serves as a dependable travel companion throughout the journey towards managing polycystic ovary syndrome (PCOS) and enhancing fertility.

In the next pages, we are going to go on a delectable trip in which we will investigate a holistic approach to wellbeing, nutrition, and fertility. Your journey is one of a kind, just as your body is. We are here to help you every step of the journey, providing you with the information, resources, and mouthwatering recipes you need to feed your body, balance your hormones, and increase your chances of becoming pregnant.

Understanding PCOS and Fertility

It is essential to have a firm understanding of the fundamentals before venturing into the realm of delectable meals that are good for fertility. PCOS, or polycystic ovary syndrome, is a prevalent hormonal condition that affects a great number of people all over the world. We will solve the riddle of PCOS and throw light on this condition. If you have a complete understanding of polycystic ovary syndrome (PCOS), you will be more able to make educated decisions regarding your food and lifestyle, which will eventually help you recover control over your health and reproductive potential.

Furthermore, today we are going to delve into the complex relationship that exists between

PCOS and fertility. You will learn how PCOS can have an effect on your capacity to conceive and, more significantly, how making dietary adjustments that are specific to your needs can play a critical part in boosting your fertility and increasing the likelihood that you will have children of your own. Because of this information, you will be able to make decisions that are in your best interest and begin on your road toward fertility with hope and optimism.

How This Cookbook Can Help

This cookbook is more than simply a collection of recipes; rather, it is a comprehensive guide that will change the way you think about food, your health, and your ability to have children. On the road to fertility and overall health, it may be your ally in the following ways:

- **Delicious and Nutritious Recipes:** Inside, you'll find a wide array of mouthwatering recipes carefully crafted to cater to your nutritional needs while delighting your taste buds. These recipes are not only delicious but also packed with fertility-boosting ingredients.

- **Expert Guidance:** Throughout the cookbook, you'll benefit from expert advice, tips, and explanations. We've collaborated with experienced nutritionists and healthcare professionals to ensure you have all the information you need at your fingertips.

- **Customizable Meal Plans:** To make your journey even more accessible, we've included weekly meal plans complete with grocery lists. These plans will help you take the guesswork out of meal preparation, ensuring that you stay on track with your PCOS diet goals.

- **Fertility Lifestyle Tips:** In addition to recipes, we'll delve into lifestyle practices that can enhance your fertility. From exercise routines tailored for PCOS to stress management techniques, we've got you covered.

- **Real-Life Inspiration:** Throughout the cookbook, you'll also find inspiring stories from individuals who have successfully navigated their PCOS journey and achieved their dream of conceiving. These stories offer hope and motivation, reminding you that your goal is within reach.

We hope that you will look at this cookbook as a complete resource that will assist you in feeding your body, reestablishing hormonal balance, and moving on with your goal of becoming a parent. Let's obtain better health, increase our energy, and experience the thrill of bringing a new life into the world all together by setting out on a trip together.

Chapter 1

PCOS and Fertility Unveiled

PCOS, which stands for polycystic ovary syndrome, is a condition that is famously difficult to understand despite the fact that it affects a considerable number of individuals all over the world. As we start down the road toward your greater health and happiness, as well as the possibility of creating a family of your own, it is a crucial topic for us to study because of the possible affect that it may have on a woman's capacity to conceive a child.

Demystifying PCOS: What You Need to Know

PCOS is sometimes referred to as the "silent disorder," despite the fact that its effects on the female body are everything but quiet. Despite this, PCOS is sometimes referred to as the "silent disorder." It is essential to dispel the myths around this condition in order to have a knowledge of how it may influence both your fertility and your overall health.

PCOS is characterized by a broad range of symptoms, in addition to disturbances in hormone levels. In spite of the fact that it is a rather prevalent endocrine ailment, affecting as many as one in ten women of reproductive age, the expression of the condition may vary widely from one individual to the next. PCOS is characterized by a variety of indications and symptoms, the most common of which are an irregular menstrual cycle, excessive hair growth, acne, weight gain, and the development of cysts on the ovaries. PCOS is defined by a number of indications and symptoms. On the other hand, it is vital to bear in mind that not every woman who has PCOS will have the same symptoms. This difference in symptoms may be very significant.

Even beyond the symptoms that are obvious on the surface, PCOS may have a substantial impact on the endocrine system. Insulin, androgens (male hormones), and estrogen are the primary hormones that are impacted, but the delicate balance of hormones in the body as a whole is disrupted as a result of the condition. These hormonal abnormalities may have a cascading affect on your reproductive system, raising the likelihood of irregular ovulation or anovulation (lack of ovulation), both of which may make it more difficult to conceive a child.

The good news is that polycystic ovary syndrome (PCOS) is an illness that can be treated, and with the appropriate therapy, its symptoms may be decreased. The first step in recovering control of your health and fertility that is caused by PCOS is to become aware of the precise ways in which the disease influences your body. This is the first step in regaining control of your health and fertility that is caused by PCOS.

The Connection Between PCOS and Fertility

People who have polycystic ovary syndrome (PCOS) often worry about the impact the disorder will have on their capacity to have children. Because PCOS is linked to hormonal irregularities as well as irregular ovulation, it may make it more challenging to conceive a child in women who have the condition. On the other hand, being diagnosed with polycystic ovarian syndrome (PCOS) does not exclude a woman from ever having the opportunity to become a parent in the future. If you empower yourself with the right knowledge, strategies, and support, there is still a chance that you will be able to fulfill your dream of establishing a family one day.

Infertility due to polycystic ovary syndrome (PCOS) is often caused by issues with ovulation that may range from being irregular to nonexistent. The procedure known as ovulation, in which an egg is expelled from the ovary and into the fallopian tube, is a necessary step in the journey toward getting pregnant. It is normal for a woman's chances of becoming pregnant to decrease if she does not ovulate regularly or if she never ovulates at all.

However, you should not give up hope; there are a number of fertility medicines as well as improvements in lifestyle that may dramatically increase your chances of having a child. You have options, such as medications that stimulate ovulation or in vitro fertilization (often referred to as IVF for its abbreviated form).

In furtherance of that, the primary focuses of this cookbook will be on the nutritional treatment of polycystic ovary syndrome (PCOS) and the improvement of fertility. Diet has a crucial part in the management of the hormonal irregularities that are associated with PCOS. These abnormalities are connected to the condition. By choosing the right foods to consume, you may aid in the control of your hormones, boost your insulin sensitivity, and support a healthy reproductive system in your body. The probability of you being able to successfully conceive a kid as a result of this will, in turn, increase.

Navigating the Path to Parenthood

The road that leads to parenthood may be paved with joy and filled with anticipation, but it also has the potential to throw a number of challenges in a woman's path along the way. PCOS sufferers who are traveling may find that they need to pay a little bit more attention to their surroundings and take extra safety measures. However, it is important to bear in mind that everyone's path is unique, and it is essential to approach it with a good attitude and the capacity to rapidly recover from any failures that may occur.

Within the pages of this cookbook, we will do all in our power to steer you in the correct path and provide assistance as you go. You will get access to recipes and meal plans that have been carefully created to improve your health and enhance your fertility. These recipes and meal plans are available to you. In addition to this, you will get expert counsel and lifestyle suggestions that will aid you in navigating the complexities of PCOS. Both of these things will be provided to you. In addition, we will have a conversation about the life-altering experiences of individuals who have conquered the challenges to conception created by PCOS in order to conceive a child and bring new life into the world. These individuals have been able to bring new life into the world. These folks are going to be a source of inspiration and motivation for us.

Your trip is also our adventure, and together, we will find the strategies and resources that will enhance your fertility while also enabling you to enjoy the scrumptious flavors that fuel your body. Your journey is also our journey. As a result, let's take the first step together toward a more improved and happier version of you, as well as the accomplishment of your goal of being a parent.

Chapter 2:

Building a Fertility-Focused Kitchen

You have arrived at the most important part of your PCOS diet journey: the kitchen. In the next chapter, we will go deeply into the fundamentals of establishing a kitchen that is geared for fertility. You've decided to take this route to improve your reproductive health, and as a result, your kitchen will become a haven where you can enjoy wholesome meals that are conducive to achieving your fertility objectives. Let's get started on constructing an environment that fosters achievement from the get-go.

Stocking Your Pantry for Success

Imagine that the cabinets in your kitchen are a genuine treasure trove filled with foods that enhance fertility, and that each shelf is stuffed to the brim with selections that are good for you and your family's health. The things you already have stashed away in your pantry and refrigerator will form the backbone of your PCOS-friendly eating plan. If you are attempting to have a family, here are some essential items that should be kept in your kitchen pantry:

Whole Grains: Whole grains like quinoa, brown rice, oats, and whole wheat pasta should be pantry staples. They provide complex carbohydrates and fiber, which help regulate blood sugar levels – a key factor in managing PCOS.

Legumes: Beans, lentils, and chickpeas are rich in plant-based protein and fiber, making them ideal choices for your pantry. They're also low on the glycemic index, helping maintain steady blood sugar levels.

Healthy Fats: Olive oil, avocado oil, and coconut oil are excellent sources of healthy fats. These fats support hormonal balance and are essential for fertility.

Nuts and Seeds: Almonds, walnuts, flaxseeds, chia seeds, and sunflower seeds provide essential nutrients like omega-3 fatty acids and fiber. They can be sprinkled on salads, yogurt, or incorporated into smoothies.

Herbs and Spices: Cinnamon, turmeric, and ginger can be powerful allies in your PCOS journey. They possess anti-inflammatory and insulin-regulating properties.

Canned Tomatoes: Canned tomatoes are versatile and great for making sauces, soups, and stews. They're rich in lycopene, an antioxidant linked to improved fertility.

Vinegars: Apple cider vinegar and balsamic vinegar can add flavor to dishes and aid in digestion and blood sugar control.

Protein Sources: Canned or dried fish, like tuna and salmon, can provide an easy source of omega-3 fatty acids. You can also stock up on quinoa and lean meats.

Dried Herbs and Spices: Expand your spice rack with herbs like rosemary, thyme, oregano, and spices like paprika and cumin. They'll elevate the flavors of your meals without the need for excessive salt or sugar.

Low-Glycemic Sweeteners: Opt for natural sweeteners like honey, maple syrup, and stevia for occasional indulgence without spiking blood sugar levels.

Essential Tools and Equipment

Not only does having a kitchen that is well-equipped help the process of making meals that are PCOS-friendly simpler, but it also makes the process more fun. The following is a list of some of the most important pieces of hardware and appliances that should be present in your kitchen if you are concerned about fertility:

Quality Knives: Invest in a set of sharp, high-quality knives. They make chopping and slicing a breeze, ensuring you'll be more likely to prepare fresh meals at home.

Cutting Boards: Having several cutting boards, preferably color-coded for different food groups, can prevent cross-contamination and make meal preparation more efficient.

Pots and Pans: A variety of pots and pans, including a non-stick skillet, a saucepan, and a Dutch oven, can accommodate various cooking methods.

Food Processor/Blender: These appliances are invaluable for making smoothies, soups, and sauces.

Mixing Bowls: A set of mixing bowls in different sizes will simplify meal preparation.

Measuring Cups and Spoons: Accurate measurements are essential for following recipes and portion control.

Baking Supplies: If you enjoy baking, stock up on items like baking sheets, cake pans, and muffin tins.

Grater/Zester: These tools can help you incorporate zest and grated vegetables into your dishes.

Slow Cooker: A slow cooker is a time-saving appliance for busy days. You can prepare healthy, hearty meals with minimal effort.

Digital Thermometer: Ensuring your meats are cooked to the right temperature is crucial for safety and flavor.

Quality Utensils: High-quality spatulas, tongs, and ladles make cooking and serving more convenient.

Food Storage Containers: Having a range of containers in various sizes will help you store leftovers and meal preps efficiently.

Smart Shopping Tips for Fertility-Friendly Ingredients

The ability to buy in the most time-effective manner possible is essential to properly manage a kitchen that is oriented on fertility. You may use the following helpful buying recommendations to aid you in making informed judgments when picking ingredients:

Plan Ahead: Create a weekly meal plan and shopping list based on your chosen recipes. This reduces the risk of impulse buying and ensures you have everything you need.

Shop the Perimeter: In most grocery stores, the fresh produce, lean proteins, and dairy are typically located along the perimeter. Focus on these areas for the bulk of your shopping.

Read Labels: Check the labels of packaged foods for hidden sugars, unhealthy fats, and artificial additives. Option for products with minimal processing.

Buy in Bulk: For non-perishable items like grains, legumes, and canned goods, buying in bulk can save you money in the long run.

Choose Seasonal Produce: Seasonal fruits and vegetables are often fresher and more affordable. They're also a great way to diversify your diet.

Visit the Farmers' Market: Local farmers' markets can be treasure troves of fresh, organic produce and other artisanal products. Plus, it's a chance to support local growers.

Stick to Your List: Be disciplined and stick to your shopping list. Avoid the temptation to buy unhealthy snacks or items that don't align with your PCOS diet.

Consider Online Shopping: Online grocery shopping can save time and help you resist in-store temptations.

Maintaining a diet that is fertile-friendly may be difficult, but if you are mentally and physically prepared for the challenge, you can improve your chances of having a successful pregnancy. You will be able to achieve this goal if you take the time to thoughtfully stock your pantry, outfit your cooking space with the essentials, and cultivate responsible shopping practices. Your kitchen will morph into a sanctuary that stimulates your creativity, facilitates healing, and offers you more agency as you continue to prepare meals that assist you on your road to improved health and fertility. In the chapters that follow, we'll look at how these components and approaches may be put to use by preparing a variety of scrumptious meals that are meant to enhance the health of your body and raise your fertility. These meals are designed to help you conceive naturally and have a healthier pregnancy overall.

Chapter 3:

Breakfast Bliss

Sunrise Starters for Hormonal Harmony

The concept that breakfast is the most essential meal of the day is one that is widely accepted, and it is vital to keep this idea in mind as you navigate the complex terrain of PCOS and fertility. In this chapter, we are going to begin on a quest to build breakfasts that not only titillate your taste senses but also set the scene for hormonal harmony throughout the day.

Your morning meal has to be a celebration of food, and it need to be planned in such a way that it gives your body the critical nutrients it requires. We've got you covered whether you're a fan of quick and simple alternatives or you want to take your time over a leisurely breakfast. Either way, we've got you covered.

Let's take a look at some breakfast choices that can help maintain hormonal harmony and increase your chances of becoming pregnant:

1. Energizing Smoothies

Smoothies are a delectable as well as nutritious way to get your day off to a good start. They are not only very useful, but they are also packed with components that are known to boost fertility. This is a major selling point for them. If you begin your day with a smoothie that boosts fertility, you will provide your body with a flood of nutrients that it need in order to operate in an optimal manner.

Ingredients to Supercharge Your Smoothie:

Leafy Greens: Spinach, kale, and Swiss chard are rich in folate and iron, which can help combat PCOS-related anemia and promote egg quality.

Berries: Blueberries, strawberries, and raspberries are loaded with antioxidants that combat inflammation and oxidative stress.

Greek Yogurt: Full of probiotics, Greek yogurt promotes gut health, which plays a crucial role in hormonal balance.

Flaxseeds and Chia Seeds: These seeds are rich in fiber and omega-3 fatty acids, supporting insulin sensitivity and reducing inflammation.

Macca Powder: Known as a fertility superfood, maca may help regulate hormones and improve egg quality.

2. Creative Omelets and Scrambles

Eggs are a fantastic source of protein and are packed to the gills with important nutrients, making them a great choice for your morning meal if you have PCOS. In the following paragraphs, we will study a number of imaginative recipes for omelets and scrambles that will not only satisfy your taste buds but will also give you with the building blocks that your body needs in order to maintain hormonal balance. These recipes will offer you with the building blocks that your body needs in order to maintain hormonal equilibrium.

Recipe: Spinach and Feta Omelet

Ingredients:

- 2 large eggs
- 1/4 cup of crumbled feta cheese
- 1/2 cup of fresh spinach, chopped
- 1/4 red bell pepper, diced
- Salt and pepper to taste
- A dash of olive oil for cooking

Instructions:

1. In a bowl, whisk the eggs until well beaten. Add salt and pepper to taste.
2. Heat a non-stick skillet over medium heat and add a dash of olive oil.
3. Pour the beaten eggs into the skillet.

4. As the eggs begin to set, add the chopped spinach, diced red bell pepper, and crumbled feta cheese on one half of the omelet.
5. Carefully fold the other half of the omelet over the filling.
6. Cook for another minute or two until the cheese begins to melt and the omelet is cooked through.
7. Slide the omelet onto a plate and serve with a sprinkle of fresh herbs, if desired.

Eggs are a good source of protein, and spinach is a leafy green that is high in folate and iron, so combining the two ingredients in an omelet makes for a scrumptious and healthy breakfast option.

3. Energizing Bowls

We have a variety of interesting bowls that will keep you satisfied while also allowing you to concentrate on what you're doing. Individuals who want a more filling breakfast will find that these bowls are the ideal vessel for their morning meal. These bowls, which are packed to the gills to the brim with components that support good hormone balance, will set your day off to a wonderful start and ensure that you have a productive day ahead of you.

Recipe: Quinoa Breakfast Bowl

Ingredients:

- 1/2 cup of cooked quinoa
- 1/4 cup of Greek yogurt

- 1/4 cup of mixed berries (blueberries, strawberries, or raspberries)
- 1 tablespoon of honey
- 1 tablespoon of chopped nuts (almonds, walnuts, or pecans)
- 1/2 teaspoon of ground cinnamon

Instructions:

1. Place some cooked quinoa in the bottom of a bowl to use as a foundation.

2. Place a small scoop of Greek yogurt in the middle of the dish.

3. Garnish with a colorful assortment of fresh berries.

4. Dollop some honey on top of the fruit.

5. For a satisfyingly crunchy bite, sprinkle with nuts that have been chopped.

6. Add a pinch of ground cinnamon as a finishing touch.

This quinoa breakfast dish will satisfy your cravings and keep your hormones in check at the same time. Quinoa offers critical minerals and is an excellent source of protein, while berries give antioxidants to counteract inflammation and oxidative stress. Both of these factors may contribute to poor health.

This is only the beginning of your culinary experience with a fertility-focused diet; these breakfast alternatives are just the beginning. Stay tuned as we go further into understanding the relationship between PCOS and your morning meals and as we explore additional scrumptious dishes. Your morning meal will evolve into a gratifying custom that not only fills your appetite but also bolsters your efforts to conceive along this trip.

Chapter 4:

Lunch for Hormonal Health

Lunch is an important component of our daily routine because it provides us with the chance to replenish, refresh, and make decisions that may have a big influence on the overall health of our hormones. In this chapter, we are going to go deeply into the art of constructing meals that will not only titillate your taste senses but will also help your path toward conception and hormonal balance. In this section, we are going to discuss three kinds of foods that may both satiate and invigorate you:

Wholesome Salads and Power Bowls

Salads and power bowls are not just about greens and veggies; they're a canvas for creativity and nourishment. These dishes offer a wide array of ingredients that can supercharge your fertility-focused diet.

How to Create a Fertility-Boosting Salad or Power Bowl

Step 1: Choose Your Base

To construct your meal, start with a base of leafy greens, whole grains, or legumes. These bases provide nutritional support in the form of vitamins, minerals, and fiber. There are a variety of options available, including chickpeas, lentils, kale, spinach, quinoa, and brown rice.

Step 2: Load Up on Vegetables

The more vibrant the spectrum of color, the better! Be sure to include a wide range of vegetables in your dish, such as carrots, bell peppers, cucumbers, cherry tomatoes, and beets. These vegetables provide a wide range of nutrients, as well as antioxidants.

Step 3: Add Protein

Proteins that are helpful to fertility are very necessary for maintaining hormonal equilibrium. Take into account options for lean proteins such as grilled chicken, tofu, tempeh, or nuts. Salmon is a fantastic option since it has a high concentration of omega-3 fatty acids, which are known to have a role in the regulation of hormones.

Step 4: Healthy Fats

Avocados, olive oil, and almonds are all excellent sources of these necessary healthy fats. These fats are important to the generation of hormones as well as the body's general wellness.

Step 5: Flavorful Extras

You can take your salad or power bowl to the next level by adding savory additions like fresh herbs, feta cheese, or a homemade vinaigrette to it. Not only can herbs like mint and basil give a burst of flavor to a dish, but they also help regulate hormones in the body.

Step 6: Keep It Balanced

Aim for a mixture that is well-balanced in terms of carbs, proteins, and fats. By doing so, you guarantee that your body will absorb a wide variety of nutrients, all of which are essential for maintaining healthy hormones and fertility.

Satisfying Sandwiches and Wraps

Sandwiches and wraps are two typical options for lunch, and both may easily be transformed into delectable delights that are good for one's fertility by making little adjustments. The methods that are listed below will instruct you on how to make a sandwich or wrap that will not only leave you feeling full but will also be friendly to your hormones:

Step 1: Choose Your Bread or Wrap

If you are looking for a low-carb choice, choose bread made with whole grains or whole wheat, or go for a wrap that is rich with nutrients, such as a tortilla made with whole grains or a lettuce leaf.

Step 2: Select Your Protein

When it comes to this situation, lean sources of protein are going to be your greatest buddies. Consider choices such as grilled chicken, turkey, or lean beef, as well as plant-based alternatives such as hummus, tofu, or black beans.

Step 3: Load Up on Veggies

Include a wide variety of veggies in your dish, such as lettuce, tomatoes, cucumbers, and bell peppers, to give it crispness, taste, and the critical elements that your body needs.

Step 4: Healthy Spreads

Remove the mayonnaise from your sandwich and replace it with a healthy spread such as hummus, Greek yogurt, or mashed avocado. These not only contribute to a creamier texture, but they also provide healthy fats and proteins.

Step 5: Flavor with Fresh Herbs and Spices

Add some fresh herbs and spices to your sandwich or wrap, such as basil, cilantro, oregano, and even a sprinkle of chili flakes, to give it a more robust flavor.

Nourishing Soups and Stews

On a winter day, there is nothing more satisfying than a hearty bowl of piping hot soup or stew. These foods have the potential to not only satiate you, but also keep your hormones in check. Here is how to prepare a healthy soup or stew that can aid you in your road toward having a baby:

Step 1: Start with a Flavorful Base

You may start by making a foundation by sautéing aromatic vegetables like onions, garlic, and celery in olive oil or any other healthy fat of your choosing. This offers a tasty base for your soup or stew, which you can then build upon.

Step 2: Add Lean Proteins

Choose lean proteins such as chicken and turkey, or choose for plant-based options such as lentils and beans. These proteins are necessary for the proper functioning of the hormone system.

Step 3: Pile on the Veggies

Stock up on a wide variety of veggies, including carrots, zucchini, sweet potatoes, and leafy greens, for optimal health. These vegetables are an excellent source of a wide variety of nutrients, including vitamins, minerals, and fiber.

Step 4: Spice It Up

Spices and herbs that are beneficial to fertility may be added to your soup or stew. Some examples are ginger, turmeric, and rosemary. These nutrients not only add to a more enjoyable taste, but they also help keep hormones in check.

Step 5: Don't Forget Healthy Grains

Incorporating nutritious grains into your stew, such as quinoa, brown rice, or barley, can give it more substance while also increasing the amount of fiber it contains.

Step 6: Simmer to Perfection

Give your creation some time to boil so the tastes can combine and you can be confident that everything works well together in the end product.

In this part of the book, we will examine a variety of recipes within each category, giving you the opportunity to combine and recombine elements in order to create a dish that caters to both your own preferences in terms of nutrition and your culinary preferences overall. Your decisions about what you eat for lunch are where you should start if you want to improve your hormonal health and increase your chances of becoming pregnant, and we will be here to help you through the whole process. Therefore, be ready to indulge in a scrumptious and nourishing noon meal that will not only satisfy your hunger pangs but will also nourish your body and improve your chances of becoming pregnant.

Chapter 5:

Dinner Delights

As the sun goes down and the day gives way to nighttime, it is the ideal time to eat a supper that focuses on providing nourishment and improving fertility. In this chapter, we are going to get down to the nitty gritty of your PCOS diet journey by looking at a variety of delicious supper alternatives that will not only satiate your cravings for delicious food but will also encourage hormonal balance and improve your fertility.

We have a variety of recipes that will meet all of your requirements, from main courses that include elements that increase fertility to delectable side dishes that compliment your meals to one-pot marvels that simplify your cooking routine. We hope that you will find these recipes useful. In addition to these mouthwatering recipes, we will also give in-depth instructions on how to cook these dinners. This will ensure that you are not only equipped with the necessary components but also with the knowledge to produce these delectable dishes for your evening meal.

Fertility-Promoting Main Courses

The main items you choose to eat are not only the focal point of your dinner table but also play an important part in the PCOS diet. These recipes have been meticulously crafted to include components that are well-known for their potential to enhance conception and to maintain hormone balance. Here are a few mouthwatering possibilities for the main course:

1. Grilled Salmon with Avocado Salsa:

Ingredients:

- Fresh salmon fillets
- Ripe avocados
- Cherry tomatoes
- Red onion
- Fresh cilantro
- Lime juice
- Olive oil
- Spices and seasonings

How to Make:

Prepare a marinade for the salmon by combining the olive oil, lime juice, and any other ingredients that you want.

Cook the salmon over the grill until it reaches the desired level of doneness.

To make the avocado salsa, combine lime juice, chopped cherry tomatoes, red onion, chopped cilantro, and diced avocados in a mixing bowl.

To serve, top the salmon that has been grilled with the colorful avocado salsa.

This main course will not only satisfy your taste buds, but it will also supply important omega-3 fatty acids as well as healthy fats, both of which are excellent for the health of your hormones.

2. Quinoa-Stuffed Bell Peppers:

Ingredients:

- Bell peppers
- Quinoa
- Ground turkey or tofu
- Spinach
- Tomatoes
- Garlic
- Spices and herbs

How to Make:

Cooking quinoa and sautéing either ground turkey or tofu with spinach, tomatoes, and garlic will result in a tasty stuffing that can be used in a variety of recipes.

Remove the seeds from the bell peppers and cut off the tops of the peppers.

Bake the peppers until they are fork soft after having the quinoa mixture stuffed within them.

This meal not only meets your need for a balance of protein and complex carbohydrates, but it also delivers an abundance of vitamins and minerals to support your body's natural defenses and keep you in excellent overall health. If you eat this meal, you will be able to satisfy both of these needs.

3. Lentil and Vegetable Curry:

Ingredients:

- Lentils
- Assorted vegetables
- Coconut milk
- Curry spices and seasonings
- Fresh cilantro

How to Make:

Cook the lentils until they are soft.

Create a decadent curry sauce by combining coconut milk and a wide variety of flavorful spices.

Mix a variety of veggies and lentils that have been cooked in the sauce that was made from the curry.

Simmer the veggies for the required amount of time.

Add a garnish of fresh cilantro before serving.

This main meal is excellent for vegetarians and is full with nutritional fiber, protein produced from plants, and a broad range of ingredients that encourage fertility. Vegetarians and vegans may both enjoy this cuisine.

Flavorful Side Dishes

If you are eating a savory main course, it is a great way to add some variety to your meals and improve the amount of nutrients you take in if you complement it with some delightful side dishes that you are eating at the same time. Take into consideration the following possibilities for side dishes to accompany your main course:

1. Roasted Asparagus with Lemon Zest:

Ingredients:

- Fresh asparagus spears
- Olive oil
- Lemon zest
- Spices and herbs

How to Make:

Combine olive oil, your preferred seasonings, and asparagus in a bowl.

Roast in the oven until the meat is cooked and has developed a faint crust.

Before serving, sprinkle the zest of one lemon over the dish.

This side dish will not only provide a splash of color to your dinner plate, but it will also give you an adequate dose of vitamins and antioxidants, all of which are essential for your health.

2. Cucumber and Tomato Salad:

Ingredients:

- Cucumbers
- Tomatoes
- Red onion
- Fresh dill
- Olive oil
- Balsamic vinegar

How to Make:

Cucumbers, tomatoes, and red onions should all be sliced.

Mix in some fresh dill, olive oil, and balsamic vinegar, then toss everything together.

Put it in the refrigerator so that it might become a delicious side dish.

This salad is a choice that is both hydrating and refreshing, and it is great for counteracting the richness of the meal that you will be eating as your main course because of its combination of these two characteristics.

Delectable One-Pot Wonders

Dinner preparation may be made much more quickly and easily with the help of one-pot marvels, which can provide a filling and savory meal. As an example, consider the following:

1. Fertility-Boosting Chicken and Rice Skillet:

Ingredients:

- Chicken breasts or thighs
- Brown rice
- Assorted vegetables
- Chicken broth
- Spices and herbs

How to Make:

To get a golden brown color, sear the chicken.

In a pan, combine brown rice, veggies, and chicken broth. Stir to combine.

Keep the lid on and continue to cook over low heat until the rice is done and the chicken is fork tender.

This recipe is a one-pot miracle that mixes protein, nutritious grains, and veggies into a single dish that is simple to cook and is nutritional and soothing all at the same time.

These recipes are simply a sample of everything else that may be found in this chapter. You will be prepared to produce these evening treats that will not only pleasure your taste but will also contribute to your general health and fertility if you follow the full directions and follow the suggestions on preparation that are provided. Let's roll up our sleeves and get to work in the kitchen so that we can bring the enchantment of foods that are known to increase fertility to your table. The first step on your path to better health and increased fertility starts right here, with each delicious meal that you cook.

Chapter 6:

Snacks and Small Bites

Even while snacking has a reputation for having a negative connotation, it is important to keep in mind that it may be an important component of a healthy diet, particularly when you are trying to conceive a child despite having PCOS. This chapter is devoted to those times when you feel your energy level dipping or your taste senses yearning for something satiating to satiate their cravings. We have painstakingly put together a selection of snacks and little nibbles that will not only satisfy your cravings for delicious food but will also help you achieve your reproductive objectives. We offer everything you could possibly need, whether you're in a hurry, have a need for something sweet, or are looking to give yourself a burst of energy.

On-the-Go Fertility Snacks

Because of the hectic nature of life, there are times when you want a snack that is not only tasty but also easy to transport and consume. These portable fertility snacks are ideal for times when you are on the road or when your schedule is very packed. They are not only simple to make, but they are also intended to provide you a surge of energy as well as sustenance in a single serving.

Recipe: Energizing Trail Mix

This handmade trail mix is a veritable treasure trove of wholesome ingredients. It includes a variety of nuts, seeds, and dried fruits, providing you with a well-balanced combination of natural sugars, healthy fats, and carbohydrates that come from sources other than processed foods. It is loaded with nutrients that are proven to enhance hormonal balance and fertility and it is packed full of these minerals.

Ingredients:

- 1 cup raw almonds
- 1 cup raw walnuts
- 1/2 cup pumpkin seeds
- 1/2 cup sunflower seeds
- 1/2 cup dried goji berries
- 1/2 cup dried cranberries

- 1/2 cup dried apricots, chopped
- 1 teaspoon ground cinnamon

Instructions:

Put all of the ingredients into a large bowl and mix them together.

To ensure a thorough blending, toss the ingredients together.

Keep the trail mix in a container that seals tightly to prevent air leakage, or split it out into tiny snack-sized bags for easy portability.

This trail mix is an excellent option for those looking for a quick snack that will also increase their energy levels. Because it is high in nutrients and strong in antioxidants and important vitamins, it is a choice that is beneficial to fertility and also delights your taste buds. This makes it a win-win.

Guilt-Free Sweet Treats

Maintaining a diet that is PCOS-friendly while still indulging in some of your favorite sweets is quite doable. In the following paragraphs, we will discuss several guilt-free sweet snacks that can satisfy your appetites for dessert without jeopardizing your efforts to achieve your reproductive objectives. These sweets have been formulated to include a reduced amount of added sugars while increasing the proportion of substances that promote fertility.

Recipe: Chia Pudding with Mixed Berries

This chia pudding is a delightfully creamy treat that you can savor without feeling guilty about indulging in. Chia seeds are an excellent source of omega-3 fatty acids as well as fiber, both of which may help maintain hormonal equilibrium and normalize insulin levels. Chia seeds can be found in most health food stores.

Ingredients:

- 1/4 cup chia seeds
- 1 cup unsweetened almond milk
- 1 tablespoon honey or maple syrup (optional)
- 1/2 teaspoon vanilla extract
- 1/2 cup mixed berries (blueberries, strawberries, raspberries)
- Fresh mint leaves for garnish (optional)

Instructions:

Chia seeds, almond milk, and vanilla essence should be mixed together in a dish. Additional sugar may be added if desired.

Make sure the chia seeds are spread out evenly by giving the mixture a good stir.

For the best results, allow the mixture to thicken in the refrigerator for at least two hours, preferably overnight.

Just before serving, top the pudding with a mixture of berries, and if you'd like, garnish it with some fresh mint leaves.

This chia pudding is not only a delicious dessert, but it is also a nutritious alternative that you may choose to indulge in when you have a hankering for something sweet. It is a good source of important nutrients, which may help maintain a healthy hormonal balance and contribute to your general well-being.

Savory Snacks for Sustained Energy

These dishes will provide you with a tasty snack that will keep you energetic for the whole of the day if you find yourself in need of one. Because of the high levels of protein, fiber, and healthy fats that they contain, eating them will give you the energy you need to face any challenges life throws your way.

Recipe: Mediterranean Hummus and Veggie Platter

This hummus platter, which takes its inspiration from the Mediterranean, is not only a delicious way to snack but also a source of many beneficial nutrients. The chickpeas that are the primary component of hummus are regarded as a PCOS-friendly cuisine due to the high levels of protein and fiber that they contain.

Ingredients:

- 1 cup homemade or store-bought hummus
- 1 cucumber, sliced
- 1 red bell pepper, cut into strips
- 1 cup cherry tomatoes
- 1/2 cup baby carrots
- Kalamata olives for garnish (optional)
- Whole-grain pita bread or whole-grain crackers

Instructions:

Position the hummus so that it is in the middle of the serving dish.

Place the cherry tomatoes, cucumber slices, red bell pepper strips, and baby carrots around the center.

Include some Kalamata olives for a taste of the Mediterranean in your dish.

For dipping, serve with pita bread made with healthy grains or crackers made with whole grains.

This platter of Mediterranean hummus is a wonderful option for a savory snack that is not only tasty but also filled with nutrients. It is an ideal choice for a snack that combines the best of both worlds. It is a fantastic method to increase the amounts of veggies and healthy fats that you consume in your diet, which contributes to improved hormonal balance and general wellness.

Snacking may be a joyful experience as well as an important component of a diet for PCOS. Not only will these meals satisfy your desires, but they will also help you work toward your reproductive objectives. These snacks and small bits will keep you satiated while supporting your path toward hormonal balance and enhanced fertility. Whether you're on the move, looking for a sweet pleasure, or in need of sustained energy, these snacks and little nibbles will come in handy. Indulge in these delectables with the awareness that you are providing both your body and your aspirations with the nourishment they need.

Chapter 7:

Sweet Endings

In a world where there is no shortage of gastronomic delights, there are few things that can compare to the happiness that comes from indulging in sweet sweets. And in this chapter of your "PCOS Diet Cookbook for Fertility," we've carefully designed a variety of desserts that will not only satiate your sweet appetite but also assist your path toward enhanced fertility. We hope you enjoy these recipes! Baking with care and purpose can be a very satisfying experience, which is why these recipes are a celebration of taste, sustenance, and love. You will learn how to do this by following the instructions carefully.

Irresistible Desserts That Support Fertility

It is not necessary for indulgence and fecundity to be in direct opposition to one another. In point of fact, some of the tastiest sweets may also be filled with components that are known to increase fertility. In this section, we offer a mouthwatering selection of sweets, each of which has been thoughtfully crafted to provide pleasure to your taste buds while also providing nourishment to your body.

Fruit-Filled Bliss: Berry Parfait

Our Berry Parfait is a beautiful symphony composed of fresh berries that are rich in antioxidants, Greek yogurt that is smooth, and honey for a touch of sweetness. This mouthwatering dessert is not only a treat for your senses, but it is also a treasure trove of vitamins and minerals that may assist in maintaining a healthy hormonal balance.

How to Make a Berry Parfait:

Ingredients:

- Fresh mixed berries (strawberries, blueberries, raspberries)
- Greek yogurt
- Honey or agave nectar
- Granola (optional)

Instructions:

Prepare your mixed berries by giving them a good wash.

Greek yogurt, mixed berries, and a drizzle of honey or agave nectar should be layered in a serving glass. Honey or agave nectar may also be used.

It is up to you to keep repeating the layers.

Granola provides both texture and taste enhancement when sprinkled on top.

Take pleasure in the vivacious parfait that stimulates fertility!

Chia Seed Pudding with a Twist

A Chia Seed Pudding with a Twist Chia seeds are abundant in omega-3 fatty acids and fiber, both of which may assist in the regulation of insulin levels, which is a primary issue for those who have PCOS. Our Chia Seed Pudding is a simple dessert that is very adaptable and can be arranged in a variety of ways to suit each individual's preferences.

How to Make Chia Seed Pudding:

Ingredients:

- Chia seeds
- Almond milk (or milk of your choice)
- Vanilla extract
- Fresh fruit (e.g., mango, kiwi, or pineapple)

- Nuts or seeds (e.g., almonds or flaxseeds)

Instructions:

In a dish, combine some chia seeds, some almond milk, and a couple of drops of vanilla essence. After giving it a good stir, place the mixture in the refrigerator and let it there for a few hours or overnight, until it has thickened.

Create a parfait out of your chia pudding by layering it with fresh fruit and topping it with a sprinkling of almonds or seeds.

Savor the nutrient-dense, decadent pudding that is filled with cream and richness.

Indulgent yet Healthy Treats

There is no rule that says indulgence must always be accompanied by feelings of regret. In this part, we will introduce you to desserts that will satisfy your sweet tooth while still adhering to the PCOS diet and the reproductive objectives that you have set for yourself.

Decadent Dark Chocolate Avocado Mousse

You don't have to limit avocado to savory meals since it can also be transformed into a rich and velvety mousse. Both dark chocolate and avocado are excellent sources of healthful fats, while dark chocolate is rich in antioxidants.

How to Make Dark Chocolate Avocado Mousse:

Ingredients:

- Ripe avocados
- Dark chocolate (70% cocoa or higher)
- Maple syrup or honey
- Vanilla extract

Instructions:

Begin by melting the dark chocolate, then allowing it to cool.

Smooth as silk is the result of blending ripe avocados, melted chocolate, your preferred kind of sweetener, and a pinch of vanilla extract together in a blender.

Place in the refrigerator, then enjoy this decadent treat that is good for fertility.

Nutty Delights: Almond and Date Truffles

These date truffles are a delicious combination of the sweetness that comes from dates and the nuttiness that comes from nuts. They are a delicious dessert that can be prepared quickly and do not need any baking on the part of the cook.

How to Make Almond and Date Truffles:

Ingredients:

- Medjool dates
- Almonds
- Cocoa powder
- Vanilla extract

Instructions:

In a food processor, combine pitted Medjool dates, almonds, cocoa powder, and a drop of vanilla essence. Continue blending the ingredients until the dough becomes sticky and can be formed into little balls.

To make bite-sized truffles out of the mixture, roll it into balls.

Relax and feast your taste buds on these energizing and scrumptious snacks.

Baking with Love and Care

When it comes to making sweets, the process of producing them may be just as satisfying as relishing the finished result. This is especially true with chocolate-based delicacies. Baking with care and attention is not simply about preparing food; rather, it is about creating memories and nurturing your soul in the process.

The Art of Mindful Baking - Baking treats for family and friends may be a relaxing and soothing activity. In the following paragraphs, we are going to discuss the concept of baking with mindfulness. Learn how to infuse your baked goods with love and purpose, turning each creation into a pleasant gift for your body and spirit in the process.

Baking for Loved Ones - Getting together with loved ones over a shared passion of baking is another great method to do so. As you prepare mouthwatering delicacies, we will discuss ways in which you and your significant other, as well as other members of your family, may participate in the process, therefore fostering a feeling of community.

In this part of the book, we urge you to indulge in your desires for sweets and enjoy the pleasure of baking, all while keeping in mind your goals with respect to PCOS and the possibility of conceiving a child. Bear in mind that the journey itself is just as significant as the objective you're hoping to accomplish at the end of it. A celebration of life, love, and the bright future that you are working hard to accomplish is embodied in each and every delectable confection that you create.

You are free to either meticulously follow the instructions for the recipes that have been provided or make adjustments to them so that they better fit your preferences. In the kitchen, you should not be scared to try new things and be creative; baking should be a pleasurable activity that provides a one-of-a-kind experience for each person who does it.

Chapter 8:

Beverages That Boost Fertility

Your choice of drinks may have a big impact on how well your body is nourished and how well your hormones are balanced, both of which are important factors in improving your fertility. This chapter is all about the power of liquid nutrition, and it features a broad variety of drinks that have been formulated to boost reproductive wellbeing.

Hydration and Hormone Balance

Before we get into the exact recipes, let's first talk about how important it is to drink enough of water throughout the day. The control of hormones, the movement of nutrients, and one's general health are all dependent on adequate hydration. Dehydration may have a bad impact on your hormone balance, which is something that is particularly important for those who are coping with PCOS.

You should begin each day by consuming a glass of water at room temperature and adding a few drops of fresh lemon juice to it. This simple practice not only aids in hydration but also gets your metabolism going and provides assistance to your digestive system. It is important to maintain proper hydration throughout the day; thus, you should have a water bottle that can be reused with you so that you can guarantee you are getting enough fluids.

Now, let's take a look at a few different kinds of beverages that will not only keep you hydrated but also provide you the critical nutrients you need to maintain your fertility.

Smoothies and Drinks for Reproductive Wellness

Fertility Boosting Smoothie

Ingredients:

- 1 cup of unsweetened almond milk
- 1/2 cup of plain Greek yogurt
- 1/2 cup of mixed berries (blueberries, strawberries, raspberries)
- 1/2 ripe banana
- 1 tablespoon of flaxseeds

- 1 tablespoon of honey (optional)
- A handful of spinach (for an extra nutrient boost)

Instructions:

Put all of the ingredients in a blender and start it up.

Mix together until it is silky smooth and creamy.

Test for sweetness, and if it's not quite right, fix it by adding honey.

Pour into a glass, and then take pleasure in the fertility-enhancing benefits!

Green Tea Elixir

Green tea is well-known for both the presence of antioxidants in its leaves and the possible reproductive advantages that may be derived from drinking it.

Ingredients:

- 1 green tea bag
- 1 cup of hot (but not boiling) water
- 1/2 teaspoon of honey
- A squeeze of lemon (optional)

Instructions:

Put the tea bag with the green tea into the cup.

Tea should be served by pouring boiling water over the tea bag.

Allow it to sit for three to five minutes.

Take out the tea bag and sweeten it with honey or punch up the taste with a few drops of lemon juice.

Take a few sips of your green tea elixir while appreciating its mellow, earthy flavor and the fact that it may help increase fertility.

Herbal Teas and Infusions

Chamomile and Lavender Infusion

Lavender and chamomile are two herbs that are well-known for their relaxing effects. These features may assist in the management of stress, which is a key factor that can impair fertility.

Ingredients:

- 1 chamomile tea bag
- 1/2 teaspoon of dried lavender buds
- 1 cup of hot water
- A touch of honey (optional)

Instructions:

Put the dried lavender buds and the tea bag with the chamomile in the cup.

The boiling water should be poured over them.

Allow it to sit for between 5 and 7 minutes.

Take out the tea bag and, if you want, stir in some honey.

In order to unwind and de-stress at the end of the day, try sipping this calming infusion.

Nettle Leaf Tea

Nettle leaf may be a helpful assistance in your attempts to conceive a child due to the high concentration of critical nutrients that it contains. Nettle leaf may be found in many different plants.

Ingredients:

- 1 nettle leaf tea bag
- 1 cup of hot water
- A slice of lemon (optional)

Instructions:

Put the tea bag with the nettle leaves into the cup you'll be using.

Tea should be poured over the tea bag once it has been infused with the hot water.

The recommended time for infusion is between 5 and 7 minutes.

You can give it a reviving kick by throwing in a slice of lemon, but it's totally optional.

Nettle leaf tea is known for its nourishing effects and you should try drinking some.

These are just few of the many fertility-enhancing beverages that you might include to your diet if you have PCOS in order to increase your chances of having a healthy pregnancy and a healthy baby. Be sure to examine other options and personalize your choice of drinks to suit both your preferences and the parameters of your diet. Be sure to drink enough of water and try to include some of these other drinks into your daily routine if you want to increase your chances of becoming pregnant.

Chapter 9:

Weekly Meal Plans

We would like to take this opportunity to welcome you to a week of scrumptious, nutrient-dense meals that have been particularly tailored to increase your fertility and help you on your road toward treating PCOS. Your body need certain nutrients and a certain amount of energy on a daily basis, and we have designed a meal plan for you that is both nutritious and calorie-dense while yet maintaining a healthy balance. These meal plans are not simply about what you are eating; rather, they are about maximizing your hormonal balance and your general well-being in a holistic sense.

Day 1: Balanced Beginnings

Breakfast: Greek Yogurt Parfait

Ingredients:

- 1 cup Greek yogurt
- 1/2 cup mixed berries
- 2 tablespoons honey

Instructions:

Build your parfait by alternating layers of Greek yogurt, mixed berries, and honey in a dish or glass.

Start your day off right with a breakfast that's both fruity and creamy.

Lunch: Quinoa and Chickpea Salad

Ingredients:

- 1 cup cooked quinoa
- 1/2 cup canned chickpeas
- 1 cup diced cucumber
- 1/4 cup crumbled feta cheese

Instructions:

A bowl should be used to combine the quinoa, chickpeas, cucumber, and feta cheese.

To make the dressing, drizzle olive oil and lemon juice over the salad.

Dinner: Baked Salmon with Asparagus

Ingredients:

- 2 salmon fillets
- 1 bunch asparagus
- Olive oil, lemon, and your favorite spices

Instructions:

Arrange the salmon and the asparagus in a single layer on a baking sheet.

Olive oil should be drizzled on top, and then seasonings should be added.

Bake the salmon and asparagus until the fish is flaky and the vegetables are tender, respectively.

Snack: Almonds and Berries

Ingredients:

- Handful of almonds
- A mix of your favorite berries

Instructions:

A satisfying snack might be a handful of almonds and a small dish of assorted berries to enjoy between meals.

Day 2: Vibrant Veggies

Breakfast: Spinach and Mushroom Omelet

Ingredients:

- 3 eggs
- Handful of spinach
- Sliced mushrooms

Instructions:

Eggs should be whisked before being poured into a pan that has been preheated and greased.

After cooking, fold in half and add spinach and mushrooms to the mixture.

Lunch: Roasted Veggie Salad

Ingredients:

- A variety of your favorite veggies (e.g., bell peppers, zucchini, cherry tomatoes)
- Olive oil, balsamic vinegar, and herbs for seasoning

Instructions:

Toss olive oil, vinegar, and fresh herbs with vegetables and roast them.

Prepare as a filling salad dish.

Dinner: Grilled Chicken with Quinoa

Ingredients:

- Grilled chicken breast
- Cooked quinoa
- Steamed broccoli

Instructions:

Grill the chicken until cooked through.

Serve with quinoa and steamed broccoli on the side.

Snack: Carrot Sticks with Hummus

Ingredients:

- Fresh carrot sticks
- Hummus for dipping

Instructions:

Combine the smooth texture of hummus with the satisfying crunch of carrot sticks.

Day 3: Omega-3 Richness

Breakfast: Chia Seed Pudding

Ingredients:

- 2 tablespoons chia seeds
- 1 cup almond milk
- Fresh fruit for topping

Instructions:

Chia seeds and almond milk should be mixed together, stirred, and then stored in the refrigerator for the night.

Add some of your preferred fresh fruit on top.

Lunch: Tuna Salad

Ingredients:

- Canned tuna
- Mixed greens
- Cherry tomatoes, cucumber, and olives

Instructions:

Produce a reviving tuna salad by combining a variety of greens and vegetables.

Dinner: Stuffed Bell Peppers

Ingredients:

- Bell peppers
- Lean ground turkey
- Brown rice
- Tomato sauce

Instructions:

Make the filling with the ground turkey and rice.

Bake stuffed bell peppers until they are fork soft.

Snack: Sliced Avocado on Whole Grain Toast

Ingredients:

- Ripe avocado
- Whole grain toast

Instructions:

To make a snack that is both healthy and satisfying, spread ripe avocado over toast made with whole grains.

Day 4: Lean Protein Power

Breakfast: Protein-Packed Smoothie

Ingredients:

- Protein powder
- Banana
- Spinach

Instructions:

A protein-rich smoothie may be made by combining protein powder, banana, and spinach with water in a blender.

Lunch: Lentil Soup

Ingredients:

- Red lentils
- Vegetables and herbs

Instructions:

To make a warming soup, just simmer red lentils with a variety of veggies and herbs.

Dinner: Baked Tilapia with Steamed Broccoli

Ingredients:

- Tilapia fillets
- Lemon juice and spices
- Steamed broccoli

Instructions:

Bake some seasoned fish in the oven until it flakes, then serve it with broccoli that has been cooked.

Snack: Cottage Cheese and Pineapple

Ingredients:

- Cottage cheese
- Fresh pineapple chunks

Instructions:

A snack that is both savory and sweet may be made by serving cottage cheese with fresh pineapple pieces on top.

Day 5: Superfood Saturday

Breakfast: Superfood Oatmeal

Ingredients:

- Rolled oats
- Chia seeds, goji berries, and nuts

Instructions:

Create a healthy breakfast by combining rolled oats, chia seeds, goji berries, and almonds to make a superfood oatmeal.

Lunch: Quinoa and Black Bean Salad

Ingredients:

- Cooked quinoa
- Black beans
- Corn, red onion, and cilantro

Instructions:

A delicious and healthy salad may be made by combining quinoa, black beans, corn, red onion, and cilantro.

Dinner: Spaghetti Squash with Turkey Meatballs

Ingredients:

- Spaghetti squash
- Ground turkey
- Tomato sauce

Instructions:

Cook spaghetti squash in the oven while you make turkey meatballs to simmer in tomato sauce.

Snack: Superfood Smoothie

Ingredients:

- Kale, banana, and blueberries
- Greek yogurt and honey

Instructions:

Create a nutritious smoothie by combining kale, banana, blueberries, Greek yogurt, and honey in a blender.

Day 6: Veggie Delight

Breakfast: Veggie Scramble

Ingredients:

- Eggs
- A variety of your favorite veggies

Instructions:

For a healthy and delicious breakfast, try scrambling some eggs with some of your favorite vegetables.

Lunch: Spinach and Strawberry Salad

Ingredients:

- Fresh spinach
- Sliced strawberries
- Almonds and feta cheese

Instructions:

For a delectable salad, toss together some fresh spinach, sliced strawberries, almonds, and crumbled feta cheese.

Dinner: Grilled Portobello Mushrooms with Quinoa

Ingredients:

- Portobello mushrooms
- Quinoa with your choice of seasoning

Instructions:

Portobello mushrooms are delicious when grilled and served over quinoa that has been seasoned.

Snack: Sliced Cucumber with Hummus

Ingredients:

- Fresh cucumber slices
- Hummus for dipping

Instructions:

Complement the smooth texture of hummus with the crunch of cucumber slices.

Day 7: Rest and Recharge

Breakfast: Overnight Oats

Ingredients:

- Rolled oats
- Almond milk
- Fresh fruit and nuts for topping

Instructions:

After combining the rolled oats and almond milk the night before, in the morning you may top the mixture with fresh fruit and nuts.

Lunch: Leftovers Day

Ingredients:

- Use any leftovers from the week.

Dinner: Sweet Potato and Black Bean Tacos

Ingredients:

- Roasted sweet potato
- Black beans, diced tomatoes, and spices

Instructions:

You can make a filling for some robust tacos by roasting sweet potatoes, combining them with black beans and chopped tomatoes, and seasoning them with any spices you choose.

Snack: Guilt-Free Popcorn

Ingredients:

- Air-popped popcorn

Instructions:

Have a bowl of this healthy, air-popped popcorn and enjoy it without feeling guilty.

Grocery Lists for Stress-Free Shopping

We have prepared detailed grocery lists for each day of the week in order to make your time spent shopping even more convenient. These lists outline all of the components that you will need, guaranteeing that you will be able to swiftly get everything you need to cook these meals that are designed to increase fertility.

Day 1: Balanced Beginnings

- Greek yogurt
- Mixed berries
- Honey
- Quinoa
- Chickpeas
- Cucumber

- Feta cheese
- Salmon fillets
- Asparagus
- Almonds

Day 2: Vibrant Veggies

- Eggs
- Spinach
- Sliced mushrooms
- A variety of your favorite veggies (bell peppers, zucchini, cherry tomatoes)
- Olive oil
- Balsamic vinegar
- Herbs
- Grilled chicken breast
- Quinoa
- Steamed broccoli
- Fresh carrot sticks
- Hummus

Day 3: Omega-3 Richness

- Chia seeds
- Almond milk
- Fresh fruit (for topping)
- Canned tuna
- Mixed greens
- Cherry tomatoes
- Cucumber
- Olives
- Bell peppers
- Lean ground turkey
- Brown rice
- Tomato sauce
- Cottage cheese
- Fresh pineapple chunks

Day 4: Lean Protein Power

- Protein powder
- Banana
- Spinach
- Rolled oats
- Chia seeds
- Goji berries
- Nuts
- Red lentils
- A variety of vegetables and herbs
- Tilapia fillets
- Lemon juice and spices
- Handful of almonds

Day 5: Superfood Saturday

- Rolled oats
- Chia seeds
- Goji berries
- Nuts
- A variety of your favorite veggies (e.g., bell peppers, zucchini, cherry tomatoes)
- Black beans
- Corn
- Red onion
- Cilantro
- Spaghetti squash
- Ground turkey
- Tomato sauce
- Kale
- Blueberries
- Greek yogurt
- Honey

Day 6: Veggie Delight

- Eggs
- A variety of your favorite veggies
- Fresh spinach
- Sliced strawberries
- Almonds
- Feta cheese
- Portobello mushrooms
- Quinoa
- Cucumber
- Hummus

Day 7: Rest and Recharge

- Rolled oats
- Almond milk
- Fresh fruit (for topping)
- Sweet potatoes
- Black beans
- Diced tomatoes
- Spices
- Air-popped popcorn

These shopping lists are meant to guarantee that you have all of the required components for each meal that you prepare during the day. You may use them as a reference when you are out shopping, which will make your experience easier and less stressful overall. I hope you enjoy your meals that will help you conceive!

Chapter 10

Fertility Lifestyle Tips

It is imperative that you take a comprehensive strategy if you want to increase your fertility while also controlling PCOS. This will help you achieve your goals more quickly. In this chapter, we will discuss three essential facets of your lifestyle that may have a significant influence on your fertility: physical activity, the management of stress, and mindful eating and self-care. Each of these facets is equally important. These components are not only independent parts of the whole; rather, they are intertwined strands that, when brought together, create a tapestry that is rich in health, well-being, and the possibility of new life. Let's go into each one of them in further detail, shall we?

Exercise and PCOS: Finding the Right Balance

Your ability to control PCOS and improve your fertility may both be significantly aided by regular exercise. However, achieving a healthy equilibrium is essential, since either excessive effort or insufficient physical exercise may lead to unfavorable outcomes in their own right. Here is the information that you need to know:

Understanding PCOS and Exercise

Polycystic ovary syndrome is often accompanied by hormonal abnormalities and insulin resistance in affected individuals. Insulin sensitivity and hormonal control are both impacted positively by regular physical activity. Regular exercise has been shown to improve your body's capacity to make efficient use of insulin, so lowering the chance of developing high blood sugar levels, which may have a negative impact on fertility. It may also assist weight control, which is beneficial for women with PCOS since these women often have an elevated risk of obesity, which can have an adverse effect on fertility.

Choosing the Right Type of Exercise

Your choice of physical activity may have a significant impact on the outcomes you get from your workouts. Jogging, swimming, and cycling are all examples of cardiovascular workouts that may help enhance insulin sensitivity and overall cardiovascular health. Building lean muscle via resistance training activities like weightlifting may aid with maintaining a healthy weight and may be beneficial for other health benefits as well. Reducing stress and enhancing relaxation are two goals that may be accomplished with the help of yoga and Pilates.

Finding the Right Balance

It is very important to choose a mode of operation that is appropriate for you. The overtraining syndrome is a condition that may be caused by excessive exercise. This condition can cause your menstrual cycle to be disrupted and can have an effect on your fertility. On the other hand, a sedentary lifestyle may lead to weight gain and exacerbate insulin resistance, both of which can have negative health consequences. Aim for consistent exercise of a moderate intensity, around 150 minutes per week, in order to enjoy the advantages of exercise without subjecting yourself to undue stress.

Stress Management and Fertility

Stress is an unavoidable aspect of contemporary life, and it may have a negative impact on your mental and physical health, as well as your ability to have children. The symptoms of polycystic ovary syndrome (PCOS) may be made worse by stress, which can also throw off a woman's menstrual cycle and prevent her from ovulating. How to handle it is as follows:

Understanding the Stress-Fertility Connection

Cortisol is known as the "stress hormone," and it is produced in your body when you are under pressure. The elevated amounts of cortisol in your body might cause a disruption in your reproductive hormones, which can result in anovulation and irregular periods. In addition, stress may influence lifestyle aspects such as sleep and food habits, which can further have an adverse effect on fertility.

Effective Stress-Reduction Techniques

The effective management of stress is essential, and there are a variety of techniques at your disposal. You may discover moments of peace by engaging in activities such as progressive muscular relaxation, deep breathing exercises, and mindfulness meditation. You may add to your arsenal of stress-relieving strategies by partaking in activities that you find enjoyable, spending time in natural settings, and cultivating and sustaining healthy social relationships.

Seeking Professional Help

Do not be afraid to seek for professional assistance if the stress you are experiencing becomes intolerable. Counseling and therapy may help you develop healthy coping mechanisms so that you can better manage the negative effects of stress and anxiety in your life. During this time spent trying to conceive a child, taking care of your emotional health is just as vital as taking care of your physical health.

Mindful Eating and Self-Care

Consuming food in a mindful manner is a habit that, over time, may alter your relationship with food, which, in turn, can improve your fertility and general well-being. Equally essential is the practice of self-care, which serves as a source of nourishment for one's mental and emotional well-being. Let's have a look at these two aspects of leading a healthy lifestyle:

The Power of Mindful Eating

Eating mindfully is giving one's complete attention to the sensory experience of eating, which includes how the meal looks, smells, tastes, and even feels in one's mouth. It encourages you to pay attention to your body's signals for hunger and fullness and to make dietary decisions that are conducive to achieving your health and reproductive objectives. The tendency to overeat, which is typical in people with PCOS, may be mitigated with the use of this technique.

Self-Care for Your Inner Self

The term "self-care" refers to more than just taking a relaxing bath or spending the day at the spa; nevertheless, these activities surely have their place. It is important to acknowledge and value your mental and emotional health in order to achieve this. Self-care methods that help you manage stress and nourish your inner self include things like keeping a journal, expressing yourself creatively, practicing mindfulness, and establishing boundaries.

The Synergy of Mindful Eating and Self-Care

When combined with other types of self-care, the practice of mindful eating creates a tremendous synergy that is impossible to achieve by itself. When you pay attention to what your body needs, you offer sustenance not just for your physical health but also for your emotional health and mental health as well. When you do this, you not only improve your physical health but also your emotional health and mental health. Your all-encompassing plan has to be regarded as a fundamental part of the approach that you are doing to achieve your goal of starting a family.

Making adjustments to one's way of life may have a significant influence on one's capacity to manage symptoms of polycystic ovary syndrome (PCOS) and to boost fertility. It is possible to pave the way for enhanced reproductive health and overall well-being by adopting a comprehensive exercise routine, establishing effective stress management skills, and embracing mindful eating and self-care practices. This may be done by preparing the body for increased fertility and overall well-being. Keep in mind that the achievement of the goal you set for yourself is not nearly as significant as the change of your whole lifestyle into one that is more conducive to your happiness and health.

Chapter 11:

Success Stories

In this uplifting chapter, we will introduce you to real-life people who have won over the hurdles of PCOS and accomplished their hopes of conception. We hope that their stories will encourage and inspire you. These astounding success stories are not only a tribute to the power of dedication and a PCOS diet personalized to the individual, but they are also a source of hope and inspiration for your own road towards fertility.

Katie's Journey: Overcoming PCOS and Embracing Motherhood

Katie's tale is one of overcoming adversity and being unflinching in one's resolve. She was in her early twenties when she received the upsetting news that she could have difficulty having a child because of her polycystic ovary syndrome (PCOS) diagnosis. This realization may have left her feeling discouraged, but instead, it drove her desire for understanding her disease and investigating natural techniques to improve her fertility. She is now able to have children.

Katie's path to pregnancy started with a steadfast determination to adhere to a diet that was PCOS-friendly. She changed her diet to include more whole foods, decreased the amount of sugar she consumed, and added fertility-enhancing components like avocado, walnuts, and lean protein to her dishes. Not only was she able to regulate the symptoms of her PCOS, but she also improved her ability to conceive a child by paying closer attention to what she ate.

She also made exercise a regular part of her routine, partaking in activities that not only assisted her in shedding extra weight but also helped lower the amount of stress she felt. In particular, she found that including yoga into her regimen was not only relaxing but also gave her a sense of agency. Katie's efforts to manage her health on a holistic level by including dietary changes, physical activity, and stress reduction ultimately paid off when she learned that she was going to be a mother. She welcomed her lovely daughter into the world with tears of happiness and an amazing feeling of accomplishment.

Katie's experience exemplifies the transforming potential of adopting a PCOS diet and making committed changes to one's lifestyle. Her path teaches us that the desire of being a parent can become a reality if we have the drive, education, and the appropriate support.

Michael and Sarah's Path to Parenthood: A Couple's Triumph Over PCOS

Not just for individuals, but also for couples, the struggle with infertility may be a difficult path to travel. The tale of Michael and Sarah is one that exemplifies the power of a committed relationship and the significance of having a same goal in order to triumph over the reproductive challenges that are caused by PCOS.

After Sarah was given a diagnosis of PCOS, she and Michael, her husband, came to the conclusion that the best way to handle the situation was to work together on it. They set out on a quest for knowledge, with the goal of discovering the most effective strategies for enhancing the fertility of both couples.

They worked together to make adjustments to their diet in order to assist Sarah's efforts to control her PCOS and achieve her reproductive objectives. Together, they cooked healthy meals that were suitable for people with PCOS. They focused on using a broad variety of fruits, vegetables, lean meats, and whole grains in their dishes. Michael, who was a constant source of support for Sarah, often assumed the role of a chef, experimenting with scrumptious meals that were tailored to meet Sarah's particular dietary requirements.

likewise the pair committed to maintaining a consistent workout routine and turned it into a joint activity that served to strengthen their bond. Not only did they become routines for physical health, but they also provided chances for connection and emotional support, such as daily walks, weekend treks, and occasional dancing lessons.

They had success and failure along the way, but they did not give up and continued on their trip. They got through difficult times because to their unwavering commitment to one another and the love they had for one another. In the end, all of their hard work paid off, and Sarah was able to conceive a child. They were ecstatic, and their path to motherhood served as a powerful illustration of the transformative potential of a strong relationship, unwavering dedication, and intentional attention to one's way of life.

Amanda's Miraculous PCOS Transformation: A Story of Resilience and Hope

The path that Amanda has taken to become a mother is nothing short of a miracle. She was given a diagnosis of PCOS at an early age, and as a result, she had to deal with the difficulties of having irregular periods and hormone abnormalities. Her medical professionals first portrayed a grim image for her, leading her to believe that her only choice may be to undergo reproductive treatments.

Amanda was certain that she would exhaust all other options before turning to drastic methods like these, so she dove headfirst into the realm of PCOS control. She took matters into her own hands and became her own advocate, doing considerable study and attempting a variety of methods to her nutrition. The road that Amanda took was characterized by a thorough grasp of the PCOS disease as well as a dogged search for a remedy that was effective for her.

She started by cutting out all processed foods and refined sugars from her diet and replacing them with natural, nutrient-dense meals that helped her maintain a healthy hormonal equilibrium. Amanda learned about the tremendous influence that specific PCOS superfoods like turmeric, flaxseeds, and spearmint tea can have, and she began including these foods into her daily regimen as a result.

In addition to focusing on stress management approaches such as yoga and meditation, Amanda did this since she was aware that stress might make PCOS symptoms worse. As she moved along her path, she found comfort in these activities and saw a decrease in the amount of stress she was experiencing.

She had to put in a lot of hard work and perseverance before she was finally rewarded with the news that she was going to be a mother without resorting to any kind of reproductive therapy. Even in the face of tremendous obstacles, Amanda's story is a remarkable monument to the power of knowledge, self-advocacy, and the possibility for change. Amanda overcame all of these obstacles by advocating for herself.

The amazing stories of people and couples who successfully negotiated the hurdles of PCOS and accomplished their goals of parenting are shown by these tales, among many more, which can be found in several other sources. They are an inspiration for your own journey, illustrating that the route to conception and motherhood can be a reality if you have the correct information, make the necessary adjustments to your lifestyle, and remain firm in your commitment. As you start on

your own personal **PCOS** diet path toward greater health and the pleasure of ushering a new life into the world, let these tales to serve as a guiding light of hope for you.

Conclusion

Take a minute to reflect on how far you've gone on your journey with the PCOS diet as you flip the last page of this cookbook. Celebrate how far you've come! Because of the information you've learned and the healthy dishes you've experimented with, you now have a higher level of understanding, which has given you more strength, and your health has improved. You have taken a fantastic first step in changing not just your diet but also your total health and well-being by beginning this journey.

A celebration of your fertility and health is more than simply an acknowledgement of your accomplishments; it is also a validation of your tenacity, drive, and the ability for change that resides within you. It is a testament to the unyielding dedication you have shown in taking charge of both your health and fertility. Now is the time to be proud of the baby steps as well as the giant jumps you've made toward nourishing your body and maintaining hormonal equilibrium.

You've prepared yourself with the information and skills to manage the hurdles that PCOS may offer since you've done your research. You have mastered the art of harnessing the curative power of food, having realized that the foods you place on your plate may be a powerful ally in your struggle against PCOS and your pursuit of conception. Not only have the foods you've made thrilled your taste senses, but they have also been a crucial factor in enhancing your chances of becoming pregnant.

This celebration extends to each and every meal that you have carefully prepared, each mouthful that you have consumed mindfully, and each and every decision that you have made to promote your well-being. Your physical form is your temple, and you have given it the respect and care that it deserves throughout your life. Keep in mind that the purpose of this voyage is not only to get at a certain location; rather, it is to bring about significant growth in yourself along the route.

During this time of rejoicing, it is important to acknowledge and appreciate the little triumphs you have achieved, such as the times you choose a fertility-boosting snack over a less healthy choice, the mornings you began your day with a nutritious smoothie, and the afternoons you relished in a hormone-balancing supper. Recognize the success you've achieved, no matter how seemingly little it may be, in controlling the symptoms of PCOS and improving your fertility. This is important. Every accomplishment brings you one step closer to realizing your ambition of starting a family of your own.

Next Steps on Your PCOS Diet Path

As you come to the end of this part of your PCOS diet adventure and look forward to the future, keep in mind that this journey is not over. Your decision to lead a healthy lifestyle and work on improving your fertility is a long-term investment in your overall health and well-being. While the information in this cookbook has laid a solid foundation for you, there are still a great many more moves to make down this route.

- **Regular Check-Ins:** Continue to monitor your progress and adapt your diet as needed. Regular check-ins with your healthcare provider or a registered dietitian can provide valuable insights and adjustments to your PCOS diet plan.

- **Staying Informed:** Stay updated on the latest research and developments in

PCOS management and fertility. Knowledge is your most potent weapon, and staying informed can help you make the best choices for your unique situation.

- **Embracing Variety:** Don't hesitate to explore new recipes and ingredients. Variety in your diet ensures that you receive a broad spectrum of nutrients and keeps mealtime exciting.

- **Support and Community:** Seek out support groups or online communities of individuals on similar journeys. Sharing experiences, challenges, and triumphs with others can be immensely motivating and reassuring.

- **Mindfulness and Self-Care:** Remember that overall well-being goes beyond what's on your plate. Continue to practice mindfulness, stress management, and self-care techniques to maintain balance in your life.

- **Fertility Consultation:** If your journey hasn't yet led to the desired outcome, consider consulting a fertility specialist. They can provide personalized guidance and options to increase your chances of conception.

The journey you take with your diet to treat PCOS is one that is unique and ever-changing. The experiences of each person are unique; but, what binds us together is the will to work for a better, more prosperous future. You've armed yourself with the information and recipes included in this cookbook, which means that you can confidently manage the hurdles that PCOS presents.

Keep in mind that realizing your goal of being a parent is not out of reach as you go on with the following stages. You are able to muster the power and use the resources necessary to make it a reality. Embrace your natural fertility, take care to continue to nurture your body, and use this cookbook to serve as a consistent source of motivation and assistance as you continue on this incredible path.

We are grateful that you have chosen to include us in the journey that you are on with your PCOS diet and fertility. I pray that every day of your life is blessed with good health, unending joy, and the excitement of hearing the heartwarming cries of a new life joining the world.